Title

The Latest Discovery On Stroke Recovery And Prevention Cookbook

Subtitle

From Heart To Plate

By

Abraham Hunter

Copyright

No part of this book may be reproduced, stored, or transmitted in any form without the prior written permission from the author.

Introduction to "The Latest Discovery on Stroke Recovery and Prevention Cookbook" by Abraham Hunter

Welcome to "The Latest Discovery on Stroke Recovery and Prevention Cookbook" by Abraham Hunter. This book is a comprehensive guide designed to empower individuals with the knowledge and tools necessary to prevent strokes and aid in the recovery process for those who have already suffered from one.

Understanding Stroke

A stroke is a medical emergency that occurs when the blood supply to part of the brain is interrupted or reduced, depriving brain tissue of oxygen and nutrients. Within minutes, brain cells begin to die. The effects of a stroke can be devastating, leading to long-term disability or even death.

Types of Strokes

There are three main types of strokes:

1. **Ischemic Stroke**: This is the most common type, accounting for about 87% of all strokes. It occurs when a blood clot blocks or

narrows an artery leading to the brain.

2. **Hemorrhagic Stroke**: This type happens when a blood vessel in the brain bursts, causing blood to spill into or around the brain, creating swelling and pressure that damages brain cells.

3. **Transient Ischemic Attack (TIA)**: Often called a mini-stroke, a TIA occurs when there is a temporary decrease in blood supply to part of the brain. The symptoms are similar to those of a full stroke but typically last only a few minutes and cause no permanent damage. However,

TIAs serve as a warning for potential future strokes.

The History of Stroke

The concept of stroke dates back to ancient times, with Hippocrates describing sudden paralysis in the 5th century B.C. Over centuries, the understanding of stroke has evolved significantly. In the 17th century, the term "stroke" was coined from the Greek word "," meaning "struck down with violence." By the 20th century, medical advancements began to uncover the causes and mechanisms of strokes, leading to better diagnostic and treatment options.

My Personal Journey

I have lived with a stroke patient, witnessing firsthand the immense challenges they face. The emotional and physical toll on both the patient and their loved ones is profound. This personal experience has driven me to explore every possible avenue for effective prevention and recovery strategies, culminating in this book.

Why This Book is Essential

Given the current high risk of stroke, it is imperative to take proactive measures. This book is more than just a collection of recipes; it is a holistic approach to health. It integrates the latest scientific discoveries with practical advice to help you lead a stroke-free life or support a loved one in their recovery journey.

30-Day Menu Plan

One of the highlights of this book is the 30-day menu plan, meticulously designed to cater to the nutritional needs of stroke patients while also being delicious and easy to prepare. Each recipe is crafted to provide essential nutrients that support brain health, improve cardiovascular function, and aid in the recovery process.

 What You Will Learn

- **The Science of Stroke**: Detailed explanations of how strokes occur, their risk factors, and the latest research on stroke prevention and recovery.
- **Nutrition and Stroke**: Insights into the role of diet in stroke prevention and recovery, including the benefits of specific foods and nutrients.
- **Lifestyle Modifications**: Practical tips on how to make sustainable lifestyle changes that reduce the risk of stroke.

- **Delicious Recipes**: A collection of recipes that are not only nutritious but also appealing to the taste buds, ensuring that stroke patients enjoy their meals while benefiting from them.
- **Comprehensive 30-Day Plan**: A step-by-step guide to planning meals for a month, complete with shopping lists and preparation tips.

Conclusion

"The Latest Discovery on Stroke Recovery and Prevention Cookbook" is an indispensable resource for anyone at risk of stroke, recovering from a stroke, or caring for a stroke patient. It combines scientific knowledge with practical advice and delicious recipes to provide a complete guide to stroke prevention and recovery. By following the guidance in this book, you can significantly reduce the risk of stroke and enhance the quality of life for those recovering from it. This book is not just a cookbook; it is a lifeline for those determined to fight against the devastating impact of stroke.

Table Of Contents

Chapter One

What is Stroke?

1. Definition of Stroke:

A stroke, also known as a cerebrovascular accident (CVA), occurs when the blood supply to part of the brain is interrupted or reduced, leading to brain cell damage or death. This interruption in blood flow deprives brain tissue of oxygen and nutrients, resulting in neurological deficits.

2. Blood Supply to the Brain:

The brain relies on a constant supply of oxygen and nutrients provided by blood vessels. Arteries carry oxygen-rich blood to the brain cells, ensuring proper function.

3. Types of Strokes:
a. Ischemic Stroke: Caused by a blockage in a blood vessel supplying blood to the brain. This blockage can be due to a blood clot forming within the vessel (thrombus) or a clot traveling from elsewhere and becoming lodged in a brain vessel (embolus).
b. Hemorrhagic Stroke: Caused by the rupture of a blood vessel in

the brain, leading to bleeding into brain tissue.

4. Causes of Stroke:
   - Hypertension (high blood pressure)
      - High cholesterol levels
      - Diabetes
      - Smoking
      - Excessive alcohol consumption
      - Obesity
      - Physical inactivity
      - Family history of stroke or heart disease
      - Age
      - Gender
      - Ethnicity

5. Disruption of Blood Flow and Brain Cell Damage:
When blood flow to part of the brain is interrupted, brain cells begin to die within minutes due to the lack of oxygen and nutrients. This can result in various neurological symptoms, including weakness, numbness, speech difficulties, vision problems, and more.

6. Symptoms of Stroke:
Common symptoms of stroke include sudden onset of:
   - Weakness or numbness in the face, arm, or leg, typically on one side of the body

- Trouble speaking or understanding speech
- Confusion
- Vision problems in one or both eyes
- Difficulty walking, dizziness, loss of balance or coordination
- Severe headache with no known cause

7. Immediate Treatment:
Stroke is a medical emergency, and prompt treatment is crucial to minimize brain damage and improve outcomes. Treatment may include:
- Clot-busting medications (if ischemic stroke)

- Mechanical removal of clots
- Management of blood pressure, blood sugar, and other medical conditions
- Rehabilitation therapies

8. Impact of Environmental and Lifestyle Factors:
- Environmental factors like air pollution and limited access to healthcare can contribute to stroke risk.
- Lifestyle choices such as smoking, excessive alcohol consumption, and physical inactivity increase the risk of stroke.

9. Prevention:

Preventing strokes involves managing risk factors through lifestyle modifications and medical interventions. Strategies for stroke prevention include:

- Controlling hypertension through medication, diet, and lifestyle changes.

- Managing cholesterol levels with medication and a heart-healthy diet.

- Controlling blood sugar levels in individuals with diabetes.

- Quitting smoking.

- Limiting alcohol consumption.

- Eating a balanced diet rich in fruits, vegetables, whole grains, and lean proteins.

- Engaging in regular physical activity.

- Maintaining a healthy weight.

- Seeking medical treatment for conditions that increase stroke risk, such as atrial fibrillation or carotid artery disease.

10. Impact on Family and Emotional Health:
Stroke not only affects the individual who experiences it but also has a profound impact on their family members and caregivers. Family members may need to provide support with daily activities, transportation to medical appointments, and emotional

encouragement during the recovery process. Additionally, stroke survivors may experience emotional challenges such as depression, anxiety, frustration, and changes in mood and personality. It's important for both stroke survivors and their loved ones to seek support from healthcare professionals, support groups, and mental health resources.

11. Rehabilitation:
Rehabilitation plays a crucial role in helping stroke survivors regain lost function and improve their quality of life. Rehabilitation programs may

include physical therapy, occupational therapy, speech therapy, and cognitive therapy tailored to the individual's needs and goals. These therapies focus on improving mobility, strength, coordination, speech and language skills, and cognitive function.

12. Long-Term Care:
Some individuals may require long-term care and support following a stroke, especially if they experience significant disabilities or cognitive impairments. This may involve assistance with activities of daily living, such as bathing, dressing, and eating, as well as

ongoing medical management and monitoring of stroke risk factors.

In summary, stroke is a complex medical condition that requires prompt recognition, emergency treatment, and long-term management to minimize brain damage, maximize recovery, and reduce the risk of future strokes. Prevention efforts and support for both stroke survivors and their families are essential components of comprehensive stroke care.

Chapter Two

The history of stroke

The history of stroke, or cerebrovascular accident, traces back to ancient times. The understanding and documentation of stroke have evolved significantly over centuries. Here is a detailed, step-by-step account of the discovery and development of knowledge about stroke:

Ancient History

Ancient Egypt (around 3000 BC)

- **Edwin Smith Papyrus**: This ancient medical text, dating back to around 3000 BC, includes the earliest descriptions of what could be interpreted as stroke. Egyptian physicians observed cases of sudden paralysis and loss of sensation, but they did not fully understand the cause.

 Ancient Greece (around 400 BC)
- **Hippocrates**: Often considered the "Father of Medicine," Hippocrates of Kos (460-370 BC) provided one of the first clinical descriptions of stroke. He used the term "apoplexy," derived from the Greek word "," meaning "struck

down with violence." He noted that individuals suddenly lost consciousness and had paralysis without a clear cause.

 Middle Ages

 Avicenna (980-1037 AD)
- **The Canon of Medicine**: Persian physician Avicenna (Ibn Sina) wrote about apoplexy in his influential medical text. He recognized that it was related to sudden disruptions in the brain, although his understanding of the underlying mechanisms was still limited.

 Renaissance Period

 Andreas Vesalius (1514-1564)
- **De Humani Corporis Fabrica**: Vesalius, a pioneering anatomist, made significant advances in the understanding of human anatomy through detailed dissections. His work laid the foundation for later studies on the brain and its blood supply.

 William Harvey (1578-1657)
- **Discovery of Blood Circulation**: Harvey's discovery of the circulation of blood in 1628 provided a crucial understanding of how blood flow and vascular health are connected to conditions like stroke.

17th to 19th Centuries

 Johann Jakob Wepfer (1620-1695)
- **Observation of Blood Clots and Hemorrhage**: Swiss physician Wepfer is credited with the first detailed descriptions of the pathological differences between ischemic stroke (caused by a clot) and hemorrhagic stroke (caused by bleeding). In his work, he connected apoplexy to blockages and bleeding in the brain's blood vessels.

 Rudolf Virchow (1821-1902)
- **Virchow's Triad**: German physician Virchow identified the

three main factors that contribute to thrombosis (blood clot formation), which are central to understanding ischemic strokes. He also coined the term "thrombosis."

20th Century

Advances in Neurology
- **Detailed Classification**: Throughout the 20th century, medical advancements allowed for better classification and understanding of different types of strokes. Technological advances, including the invention of the CT scan and MRI, revolutionized stroke diagnosis and treatment.

World Health Organization (WHO)
- **Definition and Awareness**: In 1948, the WHO included stroke in its international classification of diseases, leading to greater awareness and research focus on stroke prevention, treatment, and rehabilitation.

Late 20th Century to Present

Modern Understanding
- **Treatment and Prevention**: The development of thrombolytic therapies (like tPA, tissue plasminogen activator) in the 1990s for treating ischemic stroke marked a significant milestone.

Advances in surgical techniques and preventive measures, including the management of risk factors like hypertension and high cholesterol, have improved stroke outcomes.

 Current Research
- **Ongoing Studies**: Contemporary research continues to focus on the underlying genetic, molecular, and environmental factors contributing to stroke, aiming to develop more effective treatments and prevention strategies.

Summary
The understanding of stroke has progressed from ancient

observations of sudden paralysis to a detailed comprehension of its underlying causes and treatment options. Early descriptions by Hippocrates laid the groundwork, while significant advances in anatomy, physiology, and medical technology over the centuries have refined our understanding and treatment of this complex condition.

Chapter Three

Types Of Strokes

Types and causes of ischemic stroke

Ischemic Stroke: Detailed Explanation and Causes

An ischemic stroke occurs when a blood clot obstructs or narrows an artery supplying blood to the brain, resulting in reduced blood flow and subsequent brain tissue damage. This type of stroke accounts for about 87% of all strokes. Below is a detailed, step-by-step explanation of ischemic stroke and its causes:

Types of Ischemic Stroke

1. Thrombotic Stroke
A thrombotic stroke happens when a blood clot forms in one of the brain's arteries, gradually reducing blood flow to the brain. This type is often associated with underlying conditions that cause the arteries to narrow or become blocked over time.

- **Large Vessel Thrombosis**: Involves the major arteries like the carotid or vertebral arteries.
- **Small Vessel Disease (Lacunar Stroke)**: Involves smaller, deeper arteries in the brain.

 2. Embolic Stroke
An embolic stroke occurs when a blood clot or other debris forms away from the brain—commonly in the heart—and travels through the bloodstream to lodge in narrower brain arteries.

Causes of Ischemic Stroke

A. Thrombotic Stroke Causes

1. **Atherosclerosis**
   - **Definition**: A condition where fatty deposits (plaques) build up on the inner walls of arteries.
   - **Mechanism**: These plaques can rupture, leading to the formation of a blood clot that can block blood flow to the brain.

2. **High Blood Pressure (Hypertension)**
   - **Definition**: Chronic high blood pressure can damage the inner walls of arteries, making them more susceptible to plaque buildup and clot formation.

   - **Mechanism**: The increased pressure can lead to the thickening and hardening of arteries, narrowing the passage for blood flow.

3. **Diabetes**
   - **Definition**: A metabolic disorder characterized by high blood sugar levels.
   - **Mechanism**: High blood sugar can damage blood vessels and contribute to atherosclerosis, increasing the risk of clot formation.

4. **High Cholesterol**
   - **Definition**: Elevated levels of low-density lipoprotein (LDL)

cholesterol can lead to plaque buildup in arteries.

   - **Mechanism**: Cholesterol deposits in the arteries can narrow them, making it easier for clots to form.

5. **Smoking**
   - **Definition**: Smoking damages the blood vessels and promotes the buildup of plaque.
   - **Mechanism**: Chemicals in tobacco smoke can thicken the blood and increase plaque buildup, which can lead to clot formation.

6. **Obesity**

- **Definition**: Excess body weight can contribute to several stroke risk factors, including high blood pressure, diabetes, and high cholesterol.
   - **Mechanism**: Obesity often leads to a sedentary lifestyle, poor diet, and metabolic changes that increase stroke risk.

7. **Sedentary Lifestyle**
   - **Definition**: Lack of physical activity can increase the risk of several cardiovascular risk factors.
   - **Mechanism**: Physical inactivity is linked to higher levels of cholesterol, blood pressure, and obesity, all of which can contribute

to atherosclerosis and clot formation.

B. Embolic Stroke Causes

1. **Atrial Fibrillation (AFib)**
   - **Definition**: An irregular and often rapid heart rate that can lead to poor blood flow.
   - **Mechanism**: AFib can cause blood to pool and form clots in the heart. These clots can travel to the brain, causing an embolic stroke.

2. **Heart Attack**
   - **Definition**: Damage to the heart muscle due to inadequate

blood supply (myocardial infarction).

   - **Mechanism**: A heart attack can lead to blood clots forming in the heart chambers, which can then dislodge and travel to the brain.

3. **Heart Valve Problems**
   - **Definition**: Conditions affecting the heart valves, such as stenosis or regurgitation.
   - **Mechanism**: Abnormal blood flow through damaged valves can cause clot formation, which may travel to the brain.

4. **Patent Foramen Ovale (PFO)**

- **Definition**: A hole in the heart that didn't close the way it should after birth.
- **Mechanism**: Blood clots can pass through this hole and travel to the brain, causing a stroke.

5. **Endocarditis**
- **Definition**: An infection of the heart's inner lining.
- **Mechanism**: This infection can lead to the formation of clots that may travel to the brain.

6. **Carotid Artery Disease**
- **Definition**: Narrowing of the carotid arteries, usually due to atherosclerosis.

- **Mechanism**: Plaques in the carotid arteries can rupture, forming clots that travel to the brain.

7. **Other Embolisms**
   - **Definition**: Embolisms can also result from other sources like fat particles, air bubbles, or fragments from tumors.
   - **Mechanism**: These materials can enter the bloodstream and travel to the brain, blocking blood flow.

Preventive Measures

To prevent ischemic stroke, managing these risk factors is crucial:

1. **Healthy Diet**: Emphasize fruits, vegetables, whole grains, and lean proteins while reducing saturated fats, trans fats, and cholesterol.
2. **Regular Exercise**: Engage in moderate to vigorous physical activity for at least 150 minutes per week.
3. **Blood Pressure Control**: Monitor and manage blood pressure through diet, exercise, and medication if necessary.

4. **Cholesterol Management**: Keep cholesterol levels in check with a healthy diet and medications if required.

5. **Diabetes Management**: Control blood sugar levels through diet, exercise, and medications.

6. **Avoid Smoking**: Quit smoking and avoid exposure to secondhand smoke.

7. **Moderate Alcohol Intake**: Limit alcohol consumption to moderate levels.

8. **Weight Management**: Maintain a healthy weight through a balanced diet and regular exercise.

9. **Regular Check-ups**: Keep up with regular health screenings and follow your healthcare provider's advice.

By understanding the types and causes of ischemic stroke, individuals can take proactive steps to reduce their risk and improve their overall cardiovascular health.

Thrombotic Stroke

Thrombotic Stroke: Detailed Explanation and Step-by-Step Analysis

A thrombotic stroke occurs when a blood clot (thrombus) forms in one of the arteries supplying blood to the brain. This type of stroke is often associated with underlying conditions that cause the arteries to narrow or become blocked over time. Here's a detailed, step-by-step explanation of thrombotic stroke, its causes, symptoms, diagnosis, treatment, and prevention.

Step 1: Understanding Thrombotic Stroke

Definition

A thrombotic stroke is an ischemic stroke caused by a thrombus that forms within an artery in the brain. This clot obstructs blood flow, depriving brain tissue of essential oxygen and nutrients, leading to brain cell death.

Subtypes
- **Large Vessel Thrombosis**: Involves major brain arteries like the carotid or vertebral arteries.
- **Small Vessel Thrombosis (Lacunar Stroke)**: Involves

smaller, deeper arteries within the brain.

 Step 2: Causes and Risk Factors

 Atherosclerosis
- **Definition**: A condition where fatty deposits (plaques) build up on the inner walls of arteries.
- **Mechanism**: Plaques can rupture, leading to the formation of a blood clot that can block blood flow to the brain.

 High Blood Pressure (Hypertension)
- **Definition**: Chronic high blood pressure can damage the inner walls of arteries, making them

more susceptible to plaque buildup and clot formation.
- **Mechanism**: The increased pressure leads to thickening and hardening of arteries, narrowing the passage for blood flow.

Diabetes
- **Definition**: A metabolic disorder characterized by high blood sugar levels.
- **Mechanism**: High blood sugar can damage blood vessels and contribute to atherosclerosis, increasing the risk of clot formation.

High Cholesterol
- **Definition**: Elevated levels of low-density lipoprotein (LDL)

cholesterol can lead to plaque buildup in arteries.
- **Mechanism**: Cholesterol deposits narrow arteries, making it easier for clots to form.

 Smoking
- **Definition**: Smoking damages the blood vessels and promotes plaque buildup.
- **Mechanism**: Chemicals in tobacco smoke can thicken the blood and increase plaque buildup, leading to clot formation.

 Obesity
- **Definition**: Excess body weight can contribute to several stroke risk factors, including high blood

pressure, diabetes, and high cholesterol.
- **Mechanism**: Obesity often leads to a sedentary lifestyle, poor diet, and metabolic changes that increase stroke risk.

 Sedentary Lifestyle
- **Definition**: Lack of physical activity can increase the risk of several cardiovascular risk factors.
- **Mechanism**: Physical inactivity is linked to higher levels of cholesterol, blood pressure, and obesity, all of which contribute to atherosclerosis and clot formation.

 Step 3: Symptoms of Thrombotic Stroke

- **Sudden Numbness or Weakness**: Often on one side of the body (face, arm, or leg).
- **Confusion**: Sudden difficulty speaking or understanding speech.
- **Visual Disturbances**: Sudden trouble seeing in one or both eyes.
- **Dizziness**: Loss of balance or coordination, sometimes leading to falls.
- **Severe Headache**: Especially if it occurs suddenly and has no known cause.

Step 4: Diagnosis

Initial Assessment

- **History and Physical Examination**: Evaluating the patient's medical history and conducting a neurological examination to assess symptoms.

Imaging Studies
- **Computed Tomography (CT) Scan**: Helps identify the type of stroke and locate the clot.
- **Magnetic Resonance Imaging (MRI)**: Provides detailed images of brain tissue and blood vessels, helping to identify the affected area.
- **Carotid Ultrasound**: Evaluates blood flow through the carotid arteries to detect blockages.

- **Cerebral Angiography**: Involves injecting a contrast dye into the blood vessels to visualize the arteries in the brain.

Blood Tests
- **Complete Blood Count (CBC)**: Checks for infections or blood disorders.
- **Blood Chemistry Tests**: Evaluate blood sugar and electrolyte levels.
- **Coagulation Tests**: Measure the blood's ability to clot and can help identify clotting disorders.

Step 5: Treatment

Acute Treatment

- **Intravenous Thrombolytics (tPA)**: Tissue plasminogen activator (tPA) can dissolve the blood clot if administered within 4.5 hours of stroke onset.
- **Endovascular Procedures**: Mechanical thrombectomy involves inserting a catheter to remove the clot directly from the artery. This is usually done within 6-24 hours of symptom onset.

Supportive Care
- **Medications**: Anticoagulants (blood thinners), antiplatelet drugs (like aspirin), and medications to manage blood pressure, cholesterol, and diabetes.

- **Rehabilitation**: Physical, occupational, and speech therapy to help regain lost functions and improve quality of life.

Step 6: Prevention

Lifestyle Changes
- **Healthy Diet**: Emphasize fruits, vegetables, whole grains, and lean proteins while reducing saturated fats, trans fats, and cholesterol.
- **Regular Exercise**: Engage in moderate to vigorous physical activity for at least 150 minutes per week.

- **Quit Smoking**: Stop smoking and avoid exposure to secondhand smoke.
- **Limit Alcohol**: Drink alcohol in moderation.

 Medical Management
- **Blood Pressure Control**: Monitor and manage blood pressure through diet, exercise, and medication if necessary.
- **Cholesterol Management**: Keep cholesterol levels in check with a healthy diet and medications if required.
- **Diabetes Management**: Control blood sugar levels through diet, exercise, and medications.

- **Regular Check-ups**: Keep up with regular health screenings and follow your healthcare provider's advice.

 Summary

Thrombotic strokes occur due to the formation of a blood clot within the arteries supplying blood to the brain, often as a result of atherosclerosis and other risk factors like high blood pressure, diabetes, high cholesterol, smoking, obesity, and a sedentary lifestyle. Recognizing symptoms early and seeking prompt medical treatment can significantly improve outcomes. Preventive measures, including lifestyle changes and medical management of underlying conditions, are crucial in reducing the risk of thrombotic stroke.

Embolic Stroke

Embolic Stroke: Detailed Explanation and Step-by-Step Analysis

An embolic stroke occurs when a blood clot or other debris forms away from the brain—commonly in the heart—and travels through the bloodstream to lodge in narrower brain arteries. This type of ischemic stroke results in reduced blood flow and subsequent brain tissue damage. Here's a detailed, step-by-step explanation of embolic stroke, its causes, symptoms, diagnosis, treatment, and prevention.

Step 1: Understanding Embolic Stroke

Definition

An embolic stroke is an ischemic stroke caused by an embolus—a blood clot, air bubble, fat deposit, or other debris—that travels through the bloodstream and obstructs a blood vessel in the brain, leading to tissue damage due to lack of oxygen and nutrients.

Step 2: Causes and Risk Factors

Atrial Fibrillation (AFib)

- **Definition**: An irregular and often rapid heart rate.
- **Mechanism**: AFib can cause blood to pool in the heart chambers, particularly the atria, leading to clot formation. These clots can then travel to the brain, causing an embolic stroke.

Heart Attack
- **Definition**: Damage to the heart muscle due to inadequate blood supply (myocardial infarction).
- **Mechanism**: A heart attack can lead to the formation of blood clots in the heart, which may dislodge and travel to the brain.

Heart Valve Problems
- **Definition**: Conditions affecting the heart valves, such as stenosis (narrowing) or regurgitation (leakage).
- **Mechanism**: Abnormal blood flow through damaged valves can lead to clot formation, which can then travel to the brain.

Patent Foramen Ovale (PFO)
- **Definition**: A hole in the heart that didn't close the way it should after birth.
- **Mechanism**: Blood clots can pass through this hole and travel to the brain, causing an embolic stroke.

Endocarditis
- **Definition**: An infection of the heart's inner lining (endocardium).
- **Mechanism**: This infection can lead to the formation of clots, which can then travel to the brain.

Carotid Artery Disease
- **Definition**: Narrowing of the carotid arteries, usually due to atherosclerosis.
- **Mechanism**: Plaques in the carotid arteries can rupture, leading to the formation of emboli that travel to the brain.

Other Embolisms
- **Definition**: Embolisms can also result from other sources like

fat particles, air bubbles, or fragments from tumors.

- **Mechanism**: These materials can enter the bloodstream and travel to the brain, blocking blood flow.

 Step 3: Symptoms of Embolic Stroke

- **Sudden Numbness or Weakness**: Typically on one side of the body (face, arm, or leg).
- **Sudden Confusion**: Difficulty speaking or understanding speech.
- **Visual Disturbances**: Sudden trouble seeing in one or both eyes.

- **Dizziness**: Loss of balance or coordination, sometimes leading to falls.
- **Severe Headache**: Especially if it occurs suddenly and has no known cause.

Step 4: Diagnosis

Initial Assessment
- **History and Physical Examination**: Evaluating the patient's medical history and conducting a neurological examination to assess symptoms.

Imaging Studies

- **Computed Tomography (CT) Scan**: Helps identify the type of stroke and locate the clot.
- **Magnetic Resonance Imaging (MRI)**: Provides detailed images of brain tissue and blood vessels, helping to identify the affected area.
- **Carotid Ultrasound**: Evaluates blood flow through the carotid arteries to detect blockages.
- **Cerebral Angiography**: Involves injecting a contrast dye into the blood vessels to visualize the arteries in the brain.

Cardiac Studies

- **Electrocardiogram (ECG)**: Detects heart rhythm abnormalities like atrial fibrillation.
- **Echocardiogram**: Uses ultrasound to create images of the heart, identifying structural problems and clots.
- **Holter Monitor**: A portable ECG device worn for 24-48 hours to detect intermittent arrhythmias.

 Blood Tests
- **Complete Blood Count (CBC)**: Checks for infections or blood disorders.
- **Blood Chemistry Tests**: Evaluate blood sugar and electrolyte levels.

- **Coagulation Tests**: Measure the blood's ability to clot and can help identify clotting disorders.

 Step 5: Treatment

 Acute Treatment
- **Intravenous Thrombolytics (tPA)**: Tissue plasminogen activator (tPA) can dissolve the blood clot if administered within 4.5 hours of stroke onset.
- **Endovascular Procedures**: Mechanical thrombectomy involves inserting a catheter to remove the clot directly from the artery. This is usually done within 6-24 hours of symptom onset.

Supportive Care

- **Medications**: Anticoagulants (blood thinners), antiplatelet drugs (like aspirin), and medications to manage blood pressure, cholesterol, and diabetes.
- **Rehabilitation**: Physical, occupational, and speech therapy to help regain lost functions and improve quality of life.

Step 6: Prevention

Lifestyle Changes
- **Healthy Diet**: Emphasize fruits, vegetables, whole grains, and lean proteins while reducing saturated fats, trans fats, and cholesterol.

- **Regular Exercise**: Engage in moderate to vigorous physical activity for at least 150 minutes per week.
- **Quit Smoking**: Stop smoking and avoid exposure to secondhand smoke.
- **Limit Alcohol**: Drink alcohol in moderation.

 Medical Management
- **Blood Pressure Control**: Monitor and manage blood pressure through diet, exercise, and medication if necessary.
- **Cholesterol Management**: Keep cholesterol levels in check with a healthy diet and medications if required.

- **Diabetes Management**: Control blood sugar levels through diet, exercise, and medications.
- **Heart Health**: Manage conditions like atrial fibrillation, heart valve problems, and other cardiac issues with appropriate medications and interventions.
- **Regular Check-ups**: Keep up with regular health screenings and follow your healthcare provider's advice.

Summary

Embolic strokes occur due to the formation of an embolus that travels through the bloodstream to the brain, causing a blockage in the arteries and subsequent brain tissue damage. Recognizing symptoms early and seeking prompt medical treatment can significantly improve outcomes. Preventive measures, including lifestyle changes and medical management of underlying conditions, are crucial in reducing the risk of embolic stroke.

Chapter Four

The Environmental Impact On Stroke Disease

The environment can significantly influence the risk, incidence, and recovery outcomes of stroke. Various environmental factors, including physical, social, and economic conditions, play a role in stroke prevalence and patient recovery. Here's a detailed, step-by-step look at the impact of environmental factors on stroke:

1. **Physical Environment**

a. **Air Quality**

- **Pollution**: Exposure to air pollutants (e.g., particulate matter, nitrogen dioxide) has been linked to an increased risk of stroke.
    - **Mechanism**: Pollutants can cause inflammation, oxidative stress, and endothelial dysfunction, contributing to cardiovascular diseases including stroke.

b. **Climate and Weather**
    - **Temperature Extremes**: Both high and low temperatures can increase the risk of stroke. Cold weather can raise blood pressure, while heat can lead to dehydration and blood viscosity changes.

- **Humidity**: High humidity can exacerbate cardiovascular stress and dehydration, increasing stroke risk.

c. **Noise Pollution**
- **Chronic Noise Exposure**: Long-term exposure to high levels of noise (e.g., traffic, industrial) is associated with increased blood pressure and stress, both risk factors for stroke.

2. **Socioeconomic Environment**

a. **Socioeconomic Status (SES)**
- **Income Level**: Lower income is associated with higher stroke

incidence due to limited access to healthcare, healthy foods, and safe living conditions.

- **Education Level**: Lower educational attainment is linked to poorer health literacy, less awareness of stroke risk factors, and suboptimal management of chronic conditions.

b. **Healthcare Access**

- **Availability of Services**: Access to timely and quality healthcare can significantly reduce stroke incidence and improve outcomes through preventive care and rapid intervention.

- **Health Insurance**: Lack of insurance can lead to delayed medical care and management of stroke risk factors like hypertension and diabetes.

3. **Social Environment**

a. **Social Support Networks**
   - **Family and Community Support**: Strong social networks can provide emotional support, practical help with managing health, and motivation for rehabilitation efforts post-stroke.
   - **Isolation and Loneliness**: Social isolation is a risk factor for stroke and can hinder recovery by reducing access to care and support.

b. **Neighborhood and Community**

   - **Neighborhood Safety**: Unsafe neighborhoods can limit physical activity and access to healthcare, increasing stroke risk.

   - **Community Resources**: Availability of parks, recreational facilities, and healthy food outlets promotes a healthy lifestyle and reduces stroke risk.

4. **Built Environment**

a. **Urban vs. Rural Living**

   - **Urban Areas**: Higher access to specialized healthcare services but increased exposure to pollution and noise.

- **Rural Areas**: Lower access to healthcare and emergency services, which can delay treatment and increase stroke mortality.

b. **Infrastructure and Transportation**

- **Accessibility**: Good infrastructure and public transportation improve access to healthcare facilities and resources, aiding in prevention and timely treatment of stroke.

5. **Work Environment**

a. **Occupational Stress**

- **Job Stress**: High job stress and long working hours are associated with increased stroke risk due to elevated blood pressure and unhealthy coping mechanisms like smoking.

- **Workplace Safety**: Exposure to hazardous materials and conditions at work can contribute to stroke risk.

b. **Sedentary Work**

- **Physical Inactivity**: Sedentary jobs contribute to obesity, hypertension, and diabetes, all of which are risk factors for stroke.

- **Ergonomics and Exercise Opportunities**: Workplaces that promote physical activity and provide ergonomic workstations help reduce stroke risk.

6. **Cultural Environment**

a. **Dietary Habits**
   - **Cultural Diets**: Dietary patterns influenced by cultural norms can affect stroke risk. Diets high in salt, fat, and sugar increase stroke risk, while diets rich in fruits, vegetables, and whole grains reduce it.
   - **Eating Practices**: Meal timing and portion sizes influenced by cultural practices can impact overall health and stroke risk.

b. **Health Behaviors**

   - **Smoking and Alcohol Use**: Cultural acceptance and prevalence of smoking and alcohol use significantly affect stroke risk.

   - **Exercise Habits**: Cultural attitudes towards physical activity influence individual behavior and stroke risk.

c. **Health Beliefs and Practices**

   - **Traditional Remedies**: Reliance on traditional or alternative medicine can delay seeking proper medical treatment.

   - **Health Literacy**: Cultural attitudes towards health education and literacy can influence understanding and management of stroke risk factors.

7. **Policy Environment**

a. **Public Health Policies**
 - **Preventive Measures**: Policies promoting smoking cessation, healthy eating, and physical activity can reduce stroke incidence.
 - **Healthcare Regulations**: Policies ensuring access to healthcare and affordable medications improve stroke management and outcomes.

b. **Environmental Regulations**

- **Air Quality Standards**: Regulations to reduce air pollution can lower the risk of stroke.
- **Noise Control**: Policies to control noise pollution in residential areas can help reduce associated health risks.

c. **Emergency Response Policies**

- **Stroke Centers and Protocols**: Designation of stroke centers and implementation of rapid response protocols can significantly improve treatment outcomes.
- **Public Education Campaigns**: Raising awareness about stroke symptoms and the

importance of timely treatment can improve emergency response.

8. **Impact on Recovery**

a. **Rehabilitation Services**
- **Availability and Quality**: Access to rehabilitation services, including physical therapy, occupational therapy, and speech therapy, is crucial for stroke recovery.
- **Community Programs**: Local programs offering support groups, exercise classes, and other resources enhance recovery.

b. **Home Environment**

- **Home Modifications**: Modifications such as ramps, grab bars, and adaptive equipment can facilitate a safer and more supportive environment for stroke recovery.
  - **Supportive Living Conditions**: A stable and supportive home environment promotes better recovery outcomes.

9. **Technological Environment**

a. **Telemedicine**
  - **Access to Specialists**: Telemedicine provides remote access to stroke specialists, which

is particularly beneficial in rural or underserved areas.
   - **Follow-Up Care**: Enables continuous monitoring and follow-up care, ensuring that stroke patients adhere to rehabilitation plans and receive timely interventions.

 b. **Health Information Technology**
   - **Electronic Health Records (EHRs)**: Facilitate the coordination of care among different healthcare providers, ensuring comprehensive and continuous management of stroke risk factors.

- **Mobile Health Apps**: Apps designed for stroke recovery can provide exercises, reminders for medication, and educational materials to help patients manage their condition.

c. **Assistive Technologies**

- **Wearable Devices**: Monitors for vital signs, physical activity, and medication adherence can help manage and reduce stroke risk factors.

- **Smart Home Technologies**: Devices that aid in daily living activities (e.g., voice-activated systems, automated reminders) can support stroke patients in maintaining independence and safety.

Conclusion

Environmental factors profoundly impact both the risk of stroke and the recovery process. Addressing these factors through individual actions, community initiatives, and policy changes can significantly reduce stroke incidence and improve recovery outcomes for stroke patients. A multi-faceted approach that considers the physical, socioeconomic, social, built, work, cultural, policy, and technological environments is essential for comprehensive stroke prevention and management.

Actionable Steps for Mitigating Environmental Impact:

1. **Improve Air Quality**: Advocate for policies that reduce pollution and promote clean air.
2. **Enhance Healthcare Access**: Support initiatives that provide affordable and accessible healthcare services.
3. **Promote Healthy Lifestyles**: Implement community programs that encourage physical activity, healthy eating, and smoking cessation.

4. **Strengthen Social Support Networks**: Develop community support groups and resources for stroke patients and their families.

5. **Ensure Safe Neighborhoods**: Improve infrastructure and safety in communities to promote active living.

6. **Increase Public Awareness**: Conduct educational campaigns on stroke prevention, symptoms, and the importance of rapid treatment.

7. **Leverage Technology**: Utilize telemedicine, health apps, and assistive devices to support stroke prevention and recovery.

By focusing on these areas, we can create environments that not only reduce the risk of stroke but also support effective recovery and improve the quality of life for stroke survivors.

Chapter Five

The Impact of Alcoholism on Stroke Disease

Alcohol consumption significantly influences the risk, incidence, and outcomes of stroke. The impact varies depending on the amount and pattern of alcohol intake. Here's a detailed, step-by-step examination of the impact of alcohol on stroke disease:

1. **Introduction to Stroke and Alcohol Consumption**

a. **Types of Stroke**

- **Ischemic Stroke**: Caused by a blockage in an artery supplying blood to the brain.
- **Hemorrhagic Stroke**: Caused by bleeding in or around the brain.

 b. **Alcohol Consumption Patterns**
- **Light to Moderate Drinking**: Generally defined as up to one drink per day for women and up to two drinks per day for men.
- **Heavy Drinking**: Consuming more than the moderate amount on a regular basis.
- **Binge Drinking**: Consuming a large quantity of alcohol in a short period (typically five or more

drinks for men and four or more drinks for women in about two hours).

2. **Pathophysiological Mechanisms**

a. **Blood Pressure**
   - **Hypertension**: Chronic heavy drinking raises blood pressure, a significant risk factor for both ischemic and hemorrhagic strokes.
   - **Mechanism**: Alcohol affects the central nervous system and alters the balance of hormones regulating blood pressure.

b. **Cardiovascular Effects**

- **Atrial Fibrillation**: Heavy alcohol consumption can lead to atrial fibrillation, an irregular heart rhythm that increases the risk of ischemic stroke due to embolism.
- **Cardiomyopathy**: Chronic alcohol use can weaken the heart muscle, affecting its ability to pump blood efficiently.

c. **Coagulation**
- **Blood Clotting**: Alcohol affects platelet function and the coagulation cascade, influencing the risk of clot formation or bleeding.
- **Hypercoagulability**: Moderate consumption can decrease clotting risk, while heavy

consumption increases it due to liver damage and platelet dysfunction.

d. **Lipid Profile**
   - **Cholesterol Levels**: Moderate alcohol intake can increase high-density lipoprotein (HDL) cholesterol, potentially reducing ischemic stroke risk.
   - **Triglycerides**: Heavy drinking increases triglyceride levels, contributing to atherosclerosis.

3. **Epidemiological Evidence**

a. **Risk Variation by Consumption Level**

- **Light to Moderate Drinking**: Some studies suggest that moderate drinking may have a protective effect against ischemic stroke but can still increase the risk of hemorrhagic stroke.
- **Heavy Drinking**: Strongly associated with increased risk of both ischemic and hemorrhagic strokes.

b. **Gender and Age Differences**
- **Gender**: The impact of alcohol on stroke risk can vary by gender, with women generally at higher risk from lower levels of consumption.
- **Age**: Younger individuals engaging in binge drinking are at

significant risk for stroke, whereas moderate consumption in older adults may have different effects.

4. **Impact on Stroke Risk**

a. **Ischemic Stroke**
   - **Reduced Risk with Moderate Drinking**: Some evidence indicates a lower risk with light to moderate alcohol consumption due to beneficial cardiovascular effects.
   - **Increased Risk with Heavy Drinking**: High alcohol intake increases the risk through hypertension, atrial fibrillation, and atherosclerosis.

b. **Hemorrhagic Stroke**

- **Increased Risk**: Both moderate and heavy drinking increase the risk of hemorrhagic stroke due to elevated blood pressure and weakened blood vessel walls.

5. **Impact on Stroke Outcomes**

a. **Severity of Stroke**

- **Increased Severity**: Heavy drinking is associated with more severe strokes and poorer outcomes.

- **Mortality Rates**: Higher mortality rates are observed in heavy drinkers following a stroke.

b. **Recovery and Rehabilitation**

- **Impaired Recovery**: Alcohol can interfere with rehabilitation efforts and recovery due to its effects on cognitive and physical function.
- **Complications**: Increased risk of post-stroke complications such as infections, seizures, and recurrent strokes.

6. **Public Health Implications**

a. **Preventive Strategies**
- **Education and Awareness**: Public health campaigns to educate about the risks of heavy drinking and the benefits of moderation.

- **Screening and Intervention**: Routine screening for alcohol use in healthcare settings and offering interventions for at-risk individuals.

b. **Policy Interventions**

- **Regulation and Control**: Policies to control the sale and distribution of alcohol, including minimum legal drinking age, taxation, and advertising restrictions.

- **Support Programs**: Providing access to support programs for alcohol dependency and promoting responsible drinking.

7. **Clinical Implications**

a. **Screening and Counseling**
   - **Routine Screening**: Healthcare providers should routinely screen patients for alcohol use and provide counseling on its risks.
   - **Brief Interventions**: Implement brief interventions in primary care to reduce excessive alcohol consumption.

b. **Management of Alcohol Use Disorder**
   - **Treatment Programs**: Access to comprehensive treatment programs, including behavioral therapy and medication-assisted treatment.

- **Follow-Up Care**: Ongoing support and monitoring for individuals recovering from alcohol use disorder to prevent relapse.

8. **Research Directions**

a. **Mechanistic Studies**
 - **Understanding Pathways**: Further research into the molecular and physiological mechanisms by which alcohol influences stroke risk.
 - **Dose-Response Relationships**: Detailed studies to refine understanding of how different levels and patterns of alcohol consumption affect stroke risk.

b. **Intervention Efficacy**

- **Preventive Programs**: Evaluating the effectiveness of various preventive programs and public health policies in reducing alcohol-related stroke risk.

- **Rehabilitation Strategies**: Research on tailored rehabilitation strategies for stroke patients with a history of alcohol use.

Conclusion

Alcohol consumption has a complex relationship with stroke risk and outcomes, influenced by the amount and pattern of drinking. While light to moderate drinking may offer some protective effects against ischemic stroke, heavy drinking substantially increases the risk of both ischemic and hemorrhagic strokes. Understanding these relationships helps in developing effective public health strategies and clinical interventions to reduce stroke incidence and improve recovery outcomes. Comprehensive approaches involving education, policy interventions, clinical support, and further research are essential to mitigate the risks associated with alcohol consumption and enhance stroke prevention and management.

Chapter Six

The Impact of Smoking on Stroke Disease

Smoking has a profound impact on the risk and severity of stroke, contributing to both ischemic and hemorrhagic types. Understanding the detailed mechanisms and effects of smoking on stroke can aid in prevention and management strategies. Here's a step-by-step examination of the impact of smoking on stroke disease:

1. **Introduction to Stroke and Smoking**

a. **Types of Stroke**

- **Ischemic Stroke**: Caused by a blockage in an artery supplying blood to the brain.

- **Hemorrhagic Stroke**: Caused by bleeding in or around the brain.

b. **Prevalence of Smoking**

- **Global Statistics**: Smoking is one of the leading preventable causes of morbidity and mortality worldwide.

- **Risk Factor**: Smoking is a significant risk factor for many cardiovascular diseases, including stroke.

2. **Pathophysiological Mechanisms**

a. **Atherosclerosis**
   - **Development**: Smoking accelerates the development of atherosclerosis (hardening and narrowing of the arteries) by damaging the endothelium (inner lining of blood vessels).
   - **Impact**: Atherosclerosis in cerebral arteries can lead to ischemic strokes by causing blood clots.

b. **Blood Pressure**
   - **Hypertension**: Smoking increases blood pressure, a major

risk factor for both ischemic and hemorrhagic strokes.

 - **Mechanism**: Nicotine and other chemicals in cigarettes stimulate the release of catecholamines (e.g., adrenaline), leading to vasoconstriction and increased heart rate.

 c. **Blood Clotting**

 - **Hypercoagulability**: Smoking increases the coagulability of blood, making it more prone to clot formation.

 - **Platelet Activation**: Smoking enhances platelet aggregation and activation, increasing the likelihood of clot formation.

d. **Oxidative Stress and Inflammation**

   - **Free Radicals**: Tobacco smoke introduces free radicals into the body, leading to oxidative stress.

   - **Inflammation**: Chronic inflammation from smoking contributes to endothelial dysfunction and plaque instability.

3. **Epidemiological Evidence**

a. **Increased Stroke Risk**

   - **Relative Risk**: Smokers have a significantly higher risk of stroke compared to non-smokers. The risk increases with the number of cigarettes smoked per day.

- **Gender Differences**: The increased risk is observed in both men and women, although the magnitude may vary.

 b. **Dose-Response Relationship**
   - **Light vs. Heavy Smokers**: Even light smokers have an elevated risk of stroke, but heavy smokers face a markedly higher risk.
   - **Secondhand Smoke**: Exposure to secondhand smoke also increases stroke risk, particularly in non-smokers.

 4. **Smoking Cessation and Stroke Risk Reduction**

a. **Immediate Benefits**

- **Blood Pressure Reduction**: Quitting smoking can lead to immediate reductions in blood pressure.

- **Decreased Blood Viscosity**: Blood becomes less prone to clotting shortly after smoking cessation.

b. **Long-Term Benefits**

- **Atherosclerosis Improvement**: Over time, smoking cessation slows the progression of atherosclerosis and may even lead to some regression.

- **Stroke Risk Reduction**: Former smokers experience a

gradual decrease in stroke risk, approaching the risk level of non-smokers after several years of cessation.

5. **Impact on Stroke Outcomes**

a. **Severity and Recovery**
   - **Increased Severity**: Smokers tend to have more severe strokes compared to non-smokers.
   - **Recovery**: Smoking can negatively impact recovery outcomes due to its effects on cardiovascular health and healing processes.

b. **Post-Stroke Complications**

- **Recurrent Stroke**: Continuing to smoke after a stroke increases the risk of a recurrent stroke.

- **Other Complications**: Smokers are more likely to develop other complications such as pneumonia and deep vein thrombosis (DVT) during recovery.

6. **Public Health Implications**

a. **Prevention Strategies**

- **Education and Awareness**: Public health campaigns to raise awareness about the risks of smoking and stroke.

- **Smoking Cessation Programs**: Access to resources

and support for individuals trying to quit smoking, including nicotine replacement therapies and counseling.

  b. **Policy Interventions**

   - **Tobacco Control Policies**: Implementation of policies such as smoking bans in public places, higher taxes on tobacco products, and restrictions on tobacco advertising.

   - **Supportive Environments**: Creating environments that support healthy lifestyle choices, such as smoke-free zones and access to recreational facilities.

  7. **Clinical Implications**

a. **Screening and Intervention**

- **Routine Screening**: Healthcare providers should routinely screen for smoking habits in patients and offer cessation support.

- **Intervention Programs**: Integrating smoking cessation programs into primary care and stroke rehabilitation settings.

b. **Medication Management**

- **Antihypertensive Medications**: Managing blood pressure in smokers or those who have quit to reduce stroke risk.

- **Antiplatelet Therapy**: Use of medications such as aspirin to reduce clotting risk in high-risk individuals.

8. **Research Directions**

a. **Understanding Mechanisms**
- **Molecular Studies**: Further research on the molecular mechanisms by which smoking contributes to stroke.
- **Longitudinal Studies**: Long-term studies to understand the impact of smoking cessation on stroke risk over time.

b. **Intervention Efficacy**
- **Smoking Cessation Programs**: Evaluating the effectiveness of various smoking

cessation interventions in reducing stroke risk.

- **Policy Impact**: Assessing the impact of public health policies on smoking rates and stroke incidence.

Conclusion

Smoking has a significant and multifaceted impact on stroke risk and outcomes. By understanding the mechanisms, epidemiological evidence, and benefits of smoking cessation, healthcare providers and public health officials can develop effective strategies to reduce the incidence of stroke related to smoking. Comprehensive approaches involving education, policy interventions, and clinical support are essential to mitigate the risks associated with smoking and improve stroke prevention and recovery outcomes.

Chapter Seven

Importance of Hydration In Stroke Recovery and Prevention

Hydration plays a crucial role in the management and recovery of stroke patients. Proper hydration can significantly influence the patient's overall outcome and recovery trajectory. Here's a detailed, step-by-step look at the impact of hydration on stroke patients:

1. **Understanding Stroke and Its Effects**

a. Types of Stroke

- **Ischemic Stroke**: Caused by a blockage in a blood vessel supplying blood to the brain.
- **Hemorrhagic Stroke**: Caused by bleeding in or around the brain.

b. Consequences of Stroke
  - Impaired blood flow to the brain.
  - Potential damage to brain cells.
  - Possible long-term disabilities (motor skills, speech, cognition).

2. **Hydration and Brain Health**

a. Importance of Hydration
  - Water is vital for maintaining blood volume and circulation.

- Adequate hydration ensures optimal function of the cardiovascular system, which is crucial for brain health.

b. Impact on Blood Viscosity

- Dehydration increases blood viscosity (thickness).

- Thicker blood flows more slowly and is more prone to clotting, which can exacerbate ischemic conditions.

3. **Hydration During Acute Stroke Phase**

a. Initial Assessment

- Immediate evaluation of hydration status upon hospital admission.

- Use of blood tests (e.g., blood urea nitrogen, creatinine) to assess dehydration.

b. Intravenous (IV) Fluids

- Administer IV fluids to maintain adequate blood volume and pressure.

- Monitor electrolytes and adjust fluid composition as needed.

4. **Hydration in the Post-Stroke Recovery Phase**

a. Oral Hydration

- Encourage regular intake of water and hydrating foods.

- Consider swallowing assessments as some stroke patients may have dysphagia (difficulty swallowing).

b. Monitoring Fluid Balance

- Regular monitoring of fluid intake and output.

- Adjust fluid recommendations based on the patient's condition and comorbidities (e.g., heart failure, kidney disease).

5. **Preventing Complications Through Hydration**

a. Prevention of Deep Vein Thrombosis (DVT)

- Proper hydration helps prevent the formation of blood clots in the legs, reducing the risk of DVT.

b. Reducing Risk of Secondary Stroke

- Maintaining adequate hydration helps prevent further ischemic events by ensuring blood flow remains optimal.

6. **Nutrition and Hydration**

a. Hydrating Foods
- Incorporate fruits and vegetables with high water content

(e.g., watermelon, cucumbers, oranges).

b. Balanced Diet
   - Ensure a diet that supports overall health, including adequate fiber, vitamins, and minerals, which can indirectly support hydration.

7. **Special Considerations**

a. Cognitive Impairment
   - Stroke patients with cognitive impairment might forget to drink water.
   - Caregivers should provide regular reminders and assistance.

b. Physical Limitations

- Mobility issues may limit access to water.

- Use of adaptive devices (e.g., straws, spill-proof cups) to facilitate independent drinking.

8. **Patient and Caregiver Education**

a. Importance of Hydration

- Educate patients and caregivers about the importance of maintaining hydration.

- Provide guidelines on daily water intake goals.

b. Recognizing Signs of Dehydration

- Teach signs of dehydration (e.g., dark urine, dry mouth, confusion).
- Encourage prompt response to any signs of dehydration.

9. **Long-Term Management**

a. Routine Monitoring
- Regular check-ups to monitor hydration status.
- Continual reassessment of hydration needs based on recovery progress and any changes in health status.

b. Adaptive Strategies
- Develop long-term strategies to ensure consistent hydration (e.g.,

setting alarms, using hydration apps).

By following these steps, healthcare providers can optimize the hydration status of stroke patients, thereby improving their recovery outcomes and reducing the risk of complications. Hydration is a critical aspect of stroke management, and careful attention to it can significantly enhance patient recovery and quality of life.

Chapter Eight

Alternative Hydration To Water

Ensuring adequate hydration for stroke patients is crucial, and while water is the most direct method, there are various alternative methods to maintain hydration, especially when patients face difficulties like dysphagia (difficulty swallowing) or cognitive impairments. Here's a detailed, step-by-step look at alternative hydration methods for stroke patients:

1. **Oral Hydration Alternatives**

a. **Electrolyte Solutions**

 - **Oral Rehydration Solutions (ORS)**: Contains a balanced mix of salts and sugars to promote absorption.

 - **Sports Drinks**: Contains electrolytes like sodium and potassium which help retain fluids.

b. **Hydrating Foods**

 - **Fruits**: High water content fruits like watermelon, oranges, strawberries, cucumbers, and grapes.

 - **Vegetables**: Hydrating vegetables such as cucumbers, tomatoes, lettuce, and celery.

- **Soups and Broths**: Clear broths and soups provide fluids and essential nutrients.

c. **Gelatin and Pudding**

- **Gelatin**: High water content and easy to swallow.

- **Pudding**: Provides hydration and can be fortified with additional nutrients.

d. **Smoothies and Shakes**

- **Fruit Smoothies**: Blended fruits and vegetables with water or milk.

- **Protein Shakes**: Nutrient-rich and hydrating, especially useful for patients with nutritional deficits.

2. **Enteral Hydration**

a. **Nasogastric Tube (NG Tube)**
  - **Purpose**: Used when patients are unable to swallow.
  - **Procedure**: Tube inserted through the nose into the stomach for direct delivery of fluids and nutrients.

b. **Gastrostomy Tube (G-Tube)**
  - **Purpose**: For long-term feeding and hydration.
  - **Procedure**: Tube inserted directly into the stomach through an abdominal incision.

3. **Parenteral Hydration**

a. **Intravenous (IV) Fluids**

- **Purpose**: Direct delivery of fluids into the bloodstream.

- **Indications**: Used in acute settings or when oral/enteral hydration is not feasible.

b. **Subcutaneous Fluid Infusion (Hypodermoclysis)**

- **Purpose**: Fluid delivery into the subcutaneous tissue.

- **Indications**: Used for mild to moderate dehydration, particularly in palliative care settings.

4. **Hydration Aids and Devices**

a. **Adaptive Drinking Aids**

- **Spill-Proof Cups**: Designed to prevent spills and make drinking easier.
- **Straws and Straw Cups**: Can help patients with limited mobility or those who have difficulty tilting their heads back.

b. **Thickened Liquids**
- **Purpose**: Reduce the risk of aspiration in patients with dysphagia.
- **Products**: Commercially available thickening agents can be added to beverages and broths.

5. **Monitoring and Adjusting Hydration**

a. **Regular Assessments**

- **Fluid Balance Monitoring**: Track input and output of fluids.

- **Signs of Dehydration**: Watch for dry mouth, dark urine, confusion, and low blood pressure.

b. **Individualized Hydration Plans**

- **Customize Fluid Intake**: Based on the patient's condition, preferences, and medical needs.

- **Adjust as Needed**: Regularly reassess and modify the plan based on recovery progress and changes in health status.

6. **Educational and Behavioral Strategies**

a. **Patient and Caregiver Education**

- **Importance of Hydration**: Educate on the benefits and necessity of maintaining hydration.

- **Recognizing Dehydration**: Teach how to identify early signs of dehydration and how to respond.

b. **Incorporating Hydration into Daily Routine**

- **Scheduled Drinking Times**: Set specific times for fluid intake to ensure consistency.

- **Use of Hydration Reminders**: Use alarms, apps, or visual cues to remind patients to drink fluids regularly.

7. **Dietary Considerations**

a. **Incorporating Hydrating Foods into Meals**
   - **Balanced Meals**: Ensure meals are rich in hydrating foods.
   - **Snacks**: Include hydrating snacks like fruit slices, yogurt, and vegetables.

b. **Nutrient-Rich Fluids**
   - **Milk and Fortified Plant-Based Beverages**: Provide hydration along with essential nutrients like calcium and vitamins.
   - **Infused Water**: Add fruits, herbs, or cucumbers to water for enhanced flavor and appeal.

By using these alternative hydration methods, healthcare providers and caregivers can ensure that stroke patients maintain adequate hydration, which is critical for their recovery and overall health. Tailoring these strategies to individual patient needs and monitoring their effectiveness is key to successful hydration management.

Chapter Nine

Other Complications That May Follow Stroke Disease

Stroke can lead to a wide range of complications beyond the immediate neurological damage. These problems can affect various aspects of physical and mental health, significantly impacting a patient's quality of life. Here is a detailed, step-by-step examination of the potential problems that may arise in a stroke patient:

1. **Physical Complications**

a. **Paralysis and Muscle Weakness**

- **Hemiplegia**: Paralysis on one side of the body.
- **Hemiparesis**: Muscle weakness on one side of the body.
- **Impact**: Difficulty in performing daily activities, requiring physical therapy for recovery.

 b. **Spasticity and Muscle Contractures**

- **Spasticity**: Increased muscle tone leading to stiffness and involuntary muscle spasms.
- **Contractures**: Permanent tightening of muscles, tendons, or skin causing joint deformities.
- **Management**: Physical therapy, medications, and sometimes surgical interventions.

c. **Dysphagia**

 - **Swallowing Difficulties**: Risk of aspiration pneumonia due to food or liquid entering the lungs.

 - **Assessment and Treatment**: Swallowing assessments, dietary modifications, and potentially feeding tubes.

d. **Pain**

 - **Central Post-Stroke Pain**: Pain due to damage in the brain's pain-processing areas.

 - **Musculoskeletal Pain**: Pain from immobilization or changes in body mechanics.

- **Management**: Medications, physical therapy, and pain management techniques.

2. **Sensory Complications**

a. **Vision Problems**
   - **Hemianopia**: Loss of half of the visual field in both eyes.
   - **Diplopia**: Double vision.
   - **Management**: Vision therapy, compensatory strategies, and sometimes surgical intervention.

b. **Neglect and Inattention**
   - **Unilateral Neglect**: Inability to recognize one side of the body or environment.

- **Treatment**: Occupational therapy and visual scanning techniques.

3. **Cognitive Complications**

a. **Memory Loss**
- **Short-term and Long-term Memory Impairments**: Difficulty remembering recent events or retaining new information.
- **Management**: Cognitive rehabilitation and memory aids.

b. **Attention and Concentration Problems**
- **Reduced Focus**: Difficulty maintaining attention to tasks.

- **Management**: Cognitive exercises and environmental modifications.

c. **Executive Dysfunction**

- **Planning and Problem-Solving**: Impaired ability to plan, organize, and execute tasks.

- **Management**: Cognitive therapy and structured routines.

4. **Communication Complications**

a. **Aphasia**

- **Expressive Aphasia**: Difficulty in producing speech.

- **Receptive Aphasia**: Difficulty in understanding speech.

- **Global Aphasia**: Severe impairment in both understanding and producing speech.
   - **Management**: Speech therapy and communication aids.

 b. **Dysarthria**
   - **Slurred Speech**: Weakness or paralysis of the muscles used for speaking.
   - **Management**: Speech therapy and assistive communication devices.

 5. **Emotional and Psychological Complications**

 a. **Depression**

- **Prevalence**: Common in stroke survivors due to changes in brain chemistry and the psychological impact of the stroke.
- **Management**: Medications, psychotherapy, and support groups.

b. **Anxiety**
- **Causes**: Fear of recurrent stroke, changes in abilities, and uncertainty about the future.
- **Management**: Counseling, medications, and relaxation techniques.

c. **Emotional Lability**

- **Pseudobulbar Affect (PBA)**: Uncontrollable episodes of crying or laughing.
  - **Management**: Medications and behavioral strategies.

6. **Social and Behavioral Complications**

a. **Social Isolation**
  - **Impact**: Reduced social interaction due to physical limitations, communication difficulties, and emotional changes.
  - **Management**: Social support, involvement in community activities, and rehabilitation programs.

b. **Behavioral Changes**

- **Apathy**: Lack of interest or motivation.

- **Impulsivity**: Acting without thinking, leading to safety risks.

- **Management**: Behavioral therapy and environmental modifications.

7. **Secondary Medical Complications**

a. **Deep Vein Thrombosis (DVT)**

- **Risk**: Increased risk due to immobility.

- **Prevention**: Blood thinners, compression stockings, and regular movement.

b. **Pulmonary Embolism (PE)**

   - **Cause**: Blood clots traveling to the lungs from the legs.

   - **Prevention and Treatment**: Anticoagulant therapy and monitoring.

c. **Pneumonia**

   - **Aspiration Risk**: Swallowing difficulties leading to aspiration pneumonia.

   - **Prevention**: Swallowing assessments, dietary modifications, and respiratory therapy.

d. **Urinary Tract Infections (UTIs)**

- **Cause**: Catheter use and immobility.
- **Prevention**: Proper hygiene, regular catheter changes, and monitoring.

8. **Rehabilitation and Long-Term Management**

a. **Interdisciplinary Rehabilitation**
- **Team Approach**: Involving physiotherapists, occupational therapists, speech therapists, psychologists, and social workers.
- **Goals**: Maximizing functional independence, improving quality of life, and preventing complications.

b. **Assistive Devices and Home Modifications**

   - **Mobility Aids**: Walkers, wheelchairs, and orthotic devices.

   - **Home Adaptations**: Installing ramps, grab bars, and modifying bathrooms for accessibility.

c. **Ongoing Medical Care**

   - **Regular Monitoring**: Blood pressure, cholesterol levels, and diabetes management.

   - **Medications**: Antihypertensives, antiplatelets, anticoagulants, and statins.

Conclusion

Stroke can lead to numerous complications that affect physical, sensory, cognitive, emotional, social, and medical aspects of a patient's life. Comprehensive management involves a multidisciplinary approach to address these issues, emphasizing rehabilitation, support, and preventive measures to improve overall outcomes and quality of life for stroke survivors. Early intervention and continuous monitoring are crucial to mitigating the long-term impacts of stroke and enhancing recovery.

Chapter Ten

30 Days Recovery And Preventive Food, Cooking Plans And Nutritional Value

Here is a detailed step-by-step guide for preparing stroke-preventive foods, complete with their nutritional values. This plan includes meals for 30 days, focusing on foods rich in vitamins, minerals, healthy fats, lean proteins, and fiber, which are crucial for reducing stroke risk.

Week 1

Day 1

 Breakfast: Whole Oat Porridge with Blueberries

Ingredients:

- 1 cup rolled oats

- 2 cups water or milk

- 1/2 cup blueberries

- 1 tbsp honey (optional)

- 1/4 tsp cinnamon

Instructions:

1. In a pot, bring water or milk to a boil.

2. Add rolled oats and reduce heat to a simmer.

3. Cook for 5-7 minutes, stirring occasionally until the oats are tender.

4. Stir in blueberries and cinnamon.

5. Drizzle with honey if desired.

Nutritional Value (approximate per serving):
- Calories: 220
- Protein: 6g
- Carbohydrates: 44g
- Fiber: 6g
- Sugars: 10g
- Fat: 3g

Lunch: Cobb Salad
Ingredients:
- 2 cups mixed greens
- 1 hard-boiled egg (sliced)

- 1/2 avocado (sliced)
- 1/4 cup cherry tomatoes (halved)
- 1/4 cup cucumber (sliced)
- 1/4 cup cooked chicken breast (diced)
- 2 tbsp feta cheese
- 1 tbsp olive oil
- 1 tbsp balsamic vinegar

Instructions:
1. Arrange mixed greens on a plate.
2. Top with egg, avocado, cherry tomatoes, cucumber, chicken, and feta cheese.
3. Drizzle with olive oil and balsamic vinegar.

Nutritional Value (approximate per serving):
- Calories: 380
- Protein: 20g
- Carbohydrates: 12g
- Fiber: 8g
- Sugars: 5g
- Fat: 30g

 Dinner: Baked Salmon with Walnut Crust
Ingredients:
- 4 salmon filets
- 1/2 cup walnuts (finely chopped)
- 2 tbsp Dijon mustard
- 1 tbsp honey
- 1 tbsp olive oil
- Salt and pepper to taste

Instructions:

1. Preheat the oven to 375°F (190°C).

2. Mix walnuts, Dijon mustard, honey, olive oil, salt, and pepper in a bowl.

3. Spread mixture over salmon filets.

4. Place salmon on a baking sheet and bake for 15-20 minutes until cooked through.

Nutritional Value (approximate per serving):
- Calories: 420
- Protein: 30g
- Carbohydrates: 10g
- Fiber: 2g
- Sugars: 6g

- Fat: 30g

Day 2

 Breakfast: Egg White Frittata with Spinach and Cherry Tomatoes
Ingredients:
- 4 egg whites
- 1/2 cup spinach (chopped)
- 1/4 cup cherry tomatoes (halved)
- 1/4 cup onion (diced)
- 1 tbsp olive oil
- Salt and pepper to taste

Instructions:
1. Preheat the oven to 350°F (175°C).
2. In an oven-safe skillet, heat olive oil over medium heat.

3. Sauté onion until translucent.

4. Add spinach and cherry tomatoes, and cook until spinach is wilted.

5. Pour in egg whites, season with salt and pepper, and cook until edges start to set.

6. Transfer skillet to the oven and bake for 10 minutes until fully set.

Nutritional Value (approximate per serving):

- Calories: 120
- Protein: 12g
- Carbohydrates: 5g
- Fiber: 2g
- Sugars: 3g
- Fat: 7g

Lunch: Quinoa Salad with Black Beans

Ingredients:

- 1 cup cooked quinoa

- 1/2 cup black beans (rinsed and drained)

- 1/4 cup red bell pepper (diced)

- 1/4 cup corn (cooked)

- 1/4 cup red onion (diced)

- 2 tbsp cilantro (chopped)

- 1 tbsp olive oil

- 1 tbsp lime juice

- Salt and pepper to taste

Instructions:

1. In a large bowl, combine quinoa, black beans, bell pepper, corn, onion, and cilantro.

2. In a small bowl, whisk together olive oil, lime juice, salt, and pepper.

3. Pour dressing over the salad and toss to coat.

Nutritional Value (approximate per serving):
- Calories: 250
- Protein: 8g
- Carbohydrates: 40g
- Fiber: 8g
- Sugars: 3g
- Fat: 8g

 Dinner: Grilled Sea Bass with Mediterranean Salad

Ingredients:
- 4 sea bass filets

- 1 tbsp olive oil

- 1 tbsp lemon juice

- Salt and pepper to taste

- 2 cups mixed greens

- 1/2 cup cherry tomatoes (halved)

- 1/4 cup cucumber (sliced)

- 1/4 cup red onion (sliced)

- 1/4 cup feta cheese

- 1 tbsp olive oil

- 1 tbsp balsamic vinegar

Instructions:

1. Preheat the grill to medium-high heat.

2. Brush sea bass filets with olive oil and lemon juice, season with salt and pepper.

3. Grill filets for 3-4 minutes per side until cooked through.

4. In a bowl, combine mixed greens, cherry tomatoes, cucumber, red onion, and feta cheese.

5. Drizzle with olive oil and balsamic vinegar, toss to coat.

Nutritional Value (approximate per serving):
- Calories: 350
- Protein: 30g
- Carbohydrates: 12g
- Fiber: 4g
- Sugars: 5g
- Fat: 22g

Day 3

Breakfast: Green Protein Smoothie

Ingredients:

- 1 cup spinach

- 1 banana

- 1/2 avocado

- 1 cup almond milk

- 1 tbsp chia seeds

- 1 scoop protein powder (optional)

Instructions:

1. Combine all ingredients in a blender.

2. Blend until smooth.

Nutritional Value (approximate per serving):

- Calories: 300

- Protein: 15g

- Carbohydrates: 30g
- Fiber: 10g
- Sugars: 15g
- Fat: 15g

Lunch: Smoked Salmon Salad
Ingredients:
- 2 cups mixed greens
- 4 oz smoked salmon
- 1/4 cup red onion (sliced)
- 1/4 cup cucumber (sliced)
- 1/4 cup cherry tomatoes (halved)
- 1 tbsp capers
- 1 tbsp olive oil
- 1 tbsp lemon juice

Instructions:
1. Arrange mixed greens on a plate.

2. Top with smoked salmon, red onion, cucumber, cherry tomatoes, and capers.

3. Drizzle with olive oil and lemon juice.

Nutritional Value (approximate per serving):
- Calories: 250
- Protein: 20g
- Carbohydrates: 10g
- Fiber: 3g
- Sugars: 5g
- Fat: 15g

 Dinner: Whole Wheat Pasta with Broccoli and Tomato Sauce

Ingredients:
- 8 oz whole wheat pasta

- 2 cups broccoli florets
- 2 cups tomato sauce
- 1/4 cup Parmesan cheese
- 1 tbsp olive oil
- Salt and pepper to taste

Instructions:

1. Cook pasta according to package instructions.

2. Steam broccoli until tender.

3. In a pan, heat olive oil and add tomato sauce.

4. Toss cooked pasta and broccoli with the tomato sauce.

5. Serve with Parmesan cheese on top.

Nutritional Value (approximate per serving):

- Calories: 400
- Protein: 15g
- Carbohydrates: 70g
- Fiber: 10g
- Sugars: 10g
- Fat: 10g

*Day 4

Lunch: Turkey and Hummus Wrap
Ingredients:
- 1 whole wheat tortilla
- 3 slices turkey breast
- 2 tbsp hummus
- 1/4 cup spinach
- 1/4 cup cucumber (sliced)
- 1/4 cup red bell pepper (sliced)

Instructions:

1. Lay the tortilla flat and spread hummus evenly over it.

2. Layer turkey slices, spinach, cucumber, and bell pepper on top.

3. Roll the tortilla tightly and slice in half.

Nutritional Value (approximate per serving):
- Calories: 250
- Protein: 15g
- Carbohydrates: 30g
- Fiber: 5g
- Sugars: 3g
- Fat: 8g

Dinner: Grilled Chicken with Quinoa Salad

Ingredients:

- 4 chicken breasts
- 1 cup quinoa (rinsed)
- 2 cups water or chicken broth
- 1/4 cup red onion (diced)
- 1/4 cup cucumber (diced)
- 1/4 cup cherry tomatoes (halved)
- 2 tbsp parsley (chopped)
- 2 tbsp olive oil
- 1 tbsp lemon juice
- Salt and pepper to taste

Instructions:

1. Preheat the grill to medium-high heat.

2. Season chicken breasts with salt, pepper, and a drizzle of olive oil. Grill for 6-7 minutes on each side until cooked through.

3. In a pot, bring quinoa and water or broth to a boil. Reduce heat and simmer for 15 minutes until water is absorbed.

4. In a large bowl, combine cooked quinoa, red onion, cucumber, cherry tomatoes, and parsley.

5. In a small bowl, whisk together olive oil, lemon juice, salt, and pepper. Pour over quinoa salad and toss to combine.

6. Serve grilled chicken with quinoa salad on the side.

Nutritional Value (approximate per serving):
- Calories: 450
- Protein: 35g
- Carbohydrates: 40g
- Fiber: 6g
- Sugars: 4g
- Fat: 18g

Day 5

Breakfast: Greek Yogurt with Nuts and Chia Seeds
Ingredients:
- 1 cup Greek yogurt
- 1 tbsp chia seeds
- 1/4 cup mixed nuts (chopped)
- 1 tbsp honey (optional)

Instructions:
1. In a bowl, combine Greek yogurt, chia seeds, and mixed nuts.
2. Drizzle with honey if desired.

Nutritional Value (approximate per serving):
- Calories: 300
- Protein: 18g
- Carbohydrates: 20g
- Fiber: 5g
- Sugars: 12g
- Fat: 15g

Lunch: Vegetarian Wrap with Avocado and Quinoa
Ingredients:

- 1 whole wheat tortilla
- 1/2 avocado (sliced)
- 1/4 cup cooked quinoa
- 1/4 cup black beans (rinsed and drained)
- 1/4 cup red bell pepper (sliced)
- 1/4 cup baby spinach
- 1 tbsp olive oil
- 1 tbsp lime juice
- Salt and pepper to taste

Instructions:
1. Lay the tortilla flat and layer with avocado, quinoa, black beans, bell pepper, and spinach.
2. Drizzle with olive oil and lime juice, and season with salt and pepper.

3. Roll the tortilla tightly and slice in half.

Nutritional Value (approximate per serving):
- Calories: 350
- Protein: 10g
- Carbohydrates: 45g
- Fiber: 12g
- Sugars: 3g
- Fat: 15g

Dinner: Shrimp Tacos with Avocado Salsa
Ingredients:
- 12 shrimp (peeled and deveined)
- 1 tbsp olive oil
- 1/2 tsp chili powder

- 1/2 tsp cumin

- Salt and pepper to taste

- 4 small whole wheat tortillas

- 1 avocado (diced)

- 1/4 cup red onion (diced)

- 1/4 cup tomato (diced)

- 1 tbsp lime juice

- 2 tbsp cilantro (chopped)

Instructions:

1. In a bowl, toss shrimp with olive oil, chili powder, cumin, salt, and pepper.

2. Heat a skillet over medium-high heat and cook shrimp for 2-3 minutes per side until pink and opaque.

3. In another bowl, combine avocado, red onion, tomato, lime juice, and cilantro to make salsa.

4. Warm tortillas and fill each with shrimp and a spoonful of avocado salsa.

Nutritional Value (approximate per serving):
- Calories: 350
- Protein: 25g
- Carbohydrates: 30g
- Fiber: 8g
- Sugars: 3g
- Fat: 15g

Day 6

Breakfast: Oat Bran Muffins with Apple and Cinnamon

Ingredients:

- 1 cup oat bran
- 1 cup whole wheat flour
- 1/2 cup almond milk
- 1/4 cup honey
- 1/4 cup applesauce
- 1 apple (peeled and diced)
- 1 egg
- 1 tsp baking powder
- 1 tsp cinnamon
- 1/2 tsp vanilla extract
- 1/4 tsp salt

Instructions:

1. Preheat the oven to 375°F (190°C).

2. In a bowl, mix oat bran, whole wheat flour, baking powder, cinnamon, and salt.

3. In another bowl, whisk together almond milk, honey, applesauce, egg, and vanilla extract.

4. Combine wet and dry ingredients, then fold in diced apple.

5. Pour batter into a greased muffin tin and bake for 20-25 minutes until a toothpick comes out clean.

Nutritional Value (approximate per serving):
- Calories: 150
- Protein: 4g
- Carbohydrates: 30g

- Fiber: 5g
- Sugars: 12g
- Fat: 3g

Lunch: Turkey and Hummus Wrap
(Repeat from Day 4)

Dinner: Whole Wheat Pasta with
Broccoli and Tomato Sauce
(Repeat from Day 3)

Day 7

Breakfast: Whole Grain Toast with
Avocado and Fried Egg
Ingredients:
- 1 slice whole grain bread
- 1/2 avocado (mashed)

- 1 egg
- 1 tbsp olive oil
- Salt and pepper to taste
- Red pepper flakes (optional)

Instructions:

1. Toast the bread until golden brown.

2. Spread mashed avocado on toast, season with salt, pepper, and red pepper flakes if using.

3. In a skillet, heat olive oil over medium heat and fry the egg to desired doneness.

4. Place the egg on top of the avocado toast.

Nutritional Value (approximate per serving):
- Calories: 300
- Protein: 10g
- Carbohydrates: 25g
- Fiber: 7g
- Sugars: 2g
- Fat: 20g

Lunch: Quinoa Salad with Black Beans (Repeat from Day 2)

Dinner: Cod en Papillote with Cherry Tomatoes and Olives
Ingredients:
- 4 cod filets
- 1 cup cherry tomatoes (halved)
- 1/4 cup olives (sliced)

- 2 garlic cloves (minced)
- 2 tbsp olive oil
- 1 tbsp lemon juice
- Salt and pepper to taste
- Fresh parsley for garnish

Instructions:

1. Preheat the oven to 375°F (190°C).
2. Place each cod filet on a piece of parchment paper.
3. Top with cherry tomatoes, olives, garlic, olive oil, lemon juice, salt, and pepper.
4. Fold parchment paper to enclose the fish and create a sealed packet.

5. Place packets on a baking sheet and bake for 15-20 minutes until the fish is cooked through.
6. Garnish with fresh parsley before serving.

Nutritional Value (approximate per serving):
- Calories: 350
- Protein: 30g
- Carbohydrates: 8g
- Fiber: 2g
- Sugars: 2g
- Fat: 20g

<u>*Week 2*</u>

Day 8

Breakfast: Coconut and Mango Chia Pudding

Ingredients:
- 1/4 cup chia seeds
- 1 cup coconut milk
- 1/2 cup diced mango
- 1 tbsp honey (optional)

Instructions:
1. In a bowl, mix chia seeds and coconut milk.
2. Refrigerate for at least 2 hours or overnight until it thickens.

3. Top with diced mango and drizzle with honey if desired.

Nutritional Value (approximate per serving):
- Calories: 300
- Protein: 5g
- Carbohydrates: 30g
- Fiber: 10g
- Sugars: 15g
- Fat: 20g

Lunch: Smoked Salmon Salad (Repeat from Day 3)

Dinner: Shrimp Tacos with Avocado Salsa (Repeat from Day 5)

**Day 9

 Breakfast: DIY Protein Bars
Ingredients:
- 1 cup rolled oats
- 1/2 cup protein powder
- 1/2 cup almond butter
- 1/4 cup honey
- 1/4 cup dark chocolate chips
- 1/4 cup chopped nuts (optional)
- 1/4 cup dried fruit (optional)
- 1/4 cup chia seeds

Instructions:
1. In a bowl, mix rolled oats, protein powder, chocolate chips, nuts, dried fruit, and chia seeds.

2. In a small saucepan, warm almond butter and honey over low heat until smooth.

3. Pour the warm mixture over the dry ingredients and mix well.

4. Press the mixture into a lined baking pan and refrigerate for at least 1 hour until firm.

5. Cut into bars and store in the fridge.

Nutritional Value (approximate per serving):
- Calories: 250
- Protein: 10g
- Carbohydrates: 25g
- Fiber: 5g
- Sugars: 12g

- Fat: 12g

Lunch: Vegetarian Wrap with Avocado and Quinoa (Repeat from Day 5)

Dinner: Baked Salmon with Walnut Crust (Repeat from Day 1)

Day 10

Breakfast: Greek Yogurt with Nuts and Chia Seeds (Repeat from Day 5)

Lunch: Cobb Salad (Repeat from Day 1)

Dinner: Grilled Chicken with Quinoa Salad (Repeat from Day 4)

Day 11

Breakfast: Whole Oat Porridge with Blueberries (Repeat from Day 1)

Lunch: Quinoa Salad with Black Beans (Repeat from Day 2)

Dinner: Cod en Papillote with Cherry Tomatoes and Olives (Repeat from Day 7)

Day 12

Breakfast: Egg White Frittata with Spinach and Cherry Tomatoes (Repeat from Day 2)

Lunch: Smoked Salmon Salad (Repeat from Day 3)

Dinner: Whole Wheat Pasta with Broccoli and Tomato Sauce (Repeat from Day 3)

Day 13

Breakfast: Green Protein Smoothie (Repeat from Day 3)

Lunch: Turkey and Hummus Wrap (Repeat from Day 4)

Dinner: Grilled Sea Bass with Mediterranean Salad (Repeat from Day 2)

Day 14

Breakfast: Whole Wheat Pancakes with Sugar-Free Maple Syrup (Repeat from Day 4)

Lunch: Vegetarian Wrap with Avocado and Quinoa (Repeat from Day 5)

Dinner: Shrimp Tacos with Avocado Salsa (Repeat from Day 5)

<u>*Week 3*</u>

Day 15

Breakfast: Greek Yogurt with Nuts and Chia Seeds (Repeat from Day 5)

Lunch: Cobb Salad (Repeat from Day 1)

Dinner: Baked Salmon with Walnut Crust (Repeat from Day 1)

Day 16

Breakfast: Oat Bran Muffins with Apple and Cinnamon (Repeat from Day 6)

Lunch: Quinoa Salad with Black Beans (Repeat from Day 2)

Dinner: Grilled Chicken with Quinoa Salad (Repeat from Day 4)

Day 17

Breakfast: Whole Grain Toast with Avocado and Fried Egg (Repeat from Day 7)

Lunch: Smoked Salmon Salad (Repeat from Day 3)

Dinner: Cod en Papillote with Cherry Tomatoes and Olives (Repeat from Day 7)

Day 18

Breakfast: Coconut and Mango Chia Pudding (Repeat from Day 8)

Lunch: Vegetarian Wrap with Avocado and Quinoa (Repeat from Day 5)

Dinner: Shrimp Tacos with Avocado Salsa (Repeat from Day 5)

Day 19

Breakfast: DIY Protein Bars (Repeat from Day 9)

Lunch: Turkey and Hummus Wrap (Repeat from Day 4)

#I Dinner: Baked Salmon with Walnut Crust (Repeat from Day 1)

Day 20

Breakfast: Greek Yogurt with Nuts and Chia Seeds (Repeat from Day 5)

Lunch: Cobb Salad (Repeat from Day 1)

Dinner: Grilled Chicken with Quinoa Salad (Repeat from Day 4)

Day 21

Breakfast: Whole Oat Porridge with Blueberries (Repeat from Day 1)

Lunch: Quinoa Salad with Black Beans (Repeat from Day 2)

Dinner: Cod en Papillote with Cherry Tomatoes and Olives (Repeat from Day 7)

Week 4

Day 22

 Breakfast: Egg White Frittata with Spinach and Cherry Tomatoes (Repeat from Day 2)

 Lunch: Smoked Salmon Salad (Repeat from Day 3)

 Dinner: Whole Wheat Pasta with Broccoli and Tomato Sauce (Repeat from Day 3)

Day 23

Breakfast: Green Protein Smoothie (Repeat from Day 3)

Lunch: Turkey and Hummus Wrap (Repeat from Day 4)

Dinner: Grilled Sea Bass with Mediterranean Salad (Repeat from Day 2)

Day 24

Breakfast: Whole Wheat Pancakes with Sugar-Free Maple Syrup (Repeat from Day 4)

Lunch: Vegetarian Wrap with Avocado and Quinoa (Repeat from Day 5)

Dinner: Shrimp Tacos with Avocado Salsa (Repeat from Day 5)

Day 25

Breakfast: Greek Yogurt with Nuts and Chia Seeds (Repeat from Day 5)

Lunch: Cobb Salad (Repeat from Day 1)

Dinner: Baked Salmon with Walnut Crust (Repeat from Day 1)

Day 26

Breakfast: Oat Bran Muffins with Apple and Cinnamon (Repeat from Day 6)

Lunch: Quinoa Salad with Black Beans (Repeat from Day 2)

Dinner: Grilled Chicken with Quinoa Salad (Repeat from Day 4)

Day 27

Breakfast: Whole Grain Toast with Avocado and Fried Egg (Repeat from Day 7)

Lunch: Smoked Salmon Salad (Repeat from Day 3)

Dinner: Cod en Papillote with Cherry Tomatoes and Olives (Repeat from Day 7)

Day 28

Breakfast: Coconut and Mango Chia Pudding (Repeat from Day 8)

Lunch: Vegetarian Wrap with Avocado and Quinoa (Repeat from Day 5)

Dinner: Shrimp Tacos with Avocado Salsa (Repeat from Day 5)

Day 29

Breakfast: DIY Protein Bars (Repeat from Day 9)

Lunch: Turkey and Hummus Wrap (Repeat from Day 4)

Dinner: Baked Salmon with Walnut Crust (Repeat from Day 1)

Day 30

 Breakfast: Greek Yogurt with Nuts and Chia Seeds (Repeat from Day 5)

 Lunch: Cobb Salad (Repeat from Day 1)

 Dinner: Grilled Chicken with Quinoa Salad (Repeat from Day 4)

Nutritional Value Summary

Whole Oat Porridge with Blueberries

- **Calories**: 220

- **Protein**: 6g

- **Carbohydrates**: 44g

- **Fiber**: 6g

- **Sugars**: 10g

- **Fat**: 3g

Cobb Salad

- **Calories**: 380

- **Protein**: 20g

- **Carbohydrates**: 12g

- **Fiber**: 8g

- **Sugars**: 5g

- **Fat**: 30g

Baked Salmon with Walnut Crust

- **Calories**: 420

- **Protein**: 30g

- **Carbohydrates**: 10g

- **Fiber**: 2g

- **Sugars**: 6g

- **Fat**: 30g

Egg White Frittata with Spinach and Cherry Tomatoes

- **Calories**: 120

- **Protein**: 12g

- **Carbohydrates**: 5g

- **Fiber**: 2g

- **Sugars**: 3g

- **Fat**: 7g

Quinoa Salad with Black Beans

- **Calories**: 250
- **Protein**: 8g
- **Carbohydrates**: 40g
- **Fiber**: 8g
- **Sugars**: 3g
- **Fat**: 8g

Grilled Sea Bass with Mediterranean Salad

- **Calories**: 350
- **Protein**: 30g
- **Carbohydrates**: 12g
- **Fiber**: 4g
- **Sugars**: 5g
- **Fat**: 22g

Green Protein Smoothie

- **Calories**: 300
- **Protein**: 15g
- **Carbohydrates**: 30g
- **Fiber**: 10g
- **Sugars**: 15g
- **Fat**: 15g

Turkey and Hummus Wrap
- **Calories**: 250
- **Protein**: 15g
- **Carbohydrates**: 30g
- **Fiber**: 5g
- **Sugars**: 3g
- **Fat**: 8g

Grilled Chicken with Quinoa Salad
- **Calories**: 450
- **Protein**: 35g

- **Carbohydrates**: 40g
- **Fiber**: 6g
- **Sugars**: 4g

Whole Wheat Pasta with Broccoli and Tomato Sauce

- **Calories**: 350
- **Protein**: 15g
- **Carbohydrates**: 60g
- **Fiber**: 10g
- **Sugars**: 10g
- **Fat**: 8g

Smoked Salmon Salad

- **Calories**: 300
- **Protein**: 20g
- **Carbohydrates**: 10g

- **Fiber**: 4g
- **Sugars**: 5g
- **Fat**: 20g

Grilled Cod en Papillote with Cherry Tomatoes and Olives
- **Calories**: 350
- **Protein**: 30g
- **Carbohydrates**: 8g
- **Fiber**: 2g
- **Sugars**: 2g
- **Fat**: 20g

Shrimp Tacos with Avocado Salsa
- **Calories**: 350
- **Protein**: 25g
- **Carbohydrates**: 30g
- **Fiber**: 8g

- **Sugars**: 3g
- **Fat**: 15g

 Greek Yogurt with Nuts and Chia Seeds
- **Calories**: 300
- **Protein**: 18g
- **Carbohydrates**: 20g
- **Fiber**: 5g
- **Sugars**: 12g
- **Fat**: 15g

 DIY Protein Bars
- **Calories**: 250
- **Protein**: 10g
- **Carbohydrates**: 25g
- **Fiber**: 5g
- **Sugars**: 12g

- **Fat**: 12g

Vegetarian Wrap with Avocado and Quinoa
- **Calories**: 350
- **Protein**: 10g
- **Carbohydrates**: 45g
- **Fiber**: 12g
- **Sugars**: 3g
- **Fat**: 15g

Whole Grain Toast with Avocado and Fried Egg
- **Calories**: 300
- **Protein**: 10g
- **Carbohydrates**: 25g
- **Fiber**: 7g
- **Sugars**: 2g

- **Fat**: 20g

Coconut and Mango Chia Pudding
- **Calories**: 300
- **Protein**: 5g
- **Carbohydrates**: 30g
- **Fiber**: 10g
- **Sugars**: 15g
- **Fat**: 20g

Oat Bran Muffins with Apple and Cinnamon
- **Calories**: 150
- **Protein**: 4g
- **Carbohydrates**: 30g
- **Fiber**: 5g
- **Sugars**: 12g
- **Fat**: 3g

Whole Wheat Pancakes with Sugar-Free Maple Syrup

- **Calories**: 300

- **Protein**: 10g

- **Carbohydrates**: 50g

- **Fiber**: 8g

- **Sugars**: 5g

- **Fat**: 8g

This structured 30-day meal plan with repetitive recipes ensures consistency in nutritional intake, making it easier to stick to a stroke-preventive diet. Here is a brief list of some key foods included in the plan and their benefits for stroke prevention:

Key Foods and Their Benefits

1. **Oats**
   - **Nutritional Benefits**: High in soluble fiber, which helps lower cholesterol levels.
   - **Stroke Prevention**: Reduces the risk of atherosclerosis and heart disease.

2. **Leafy Greens (Spinach, Kale)**
   - **Nutritional Benefits**: Rich in folate, potassium, and magnesium.
   - **Stroke Prevention**: Lowers blood pressure and improves arterial function.

3. **Berries (Blueberries, Strawberries)**
   - **Nutritional Benefits**: High in antioxidants and fiber.
   - **Stroke Prevention**: Reduces oxidative stress and inflammation.

4. **Nuts and Seeds (Almonds, Chia Seeds)**
   - **Nutritional Benefits**: Source of healthy fats, protein, and fiber.
   - **Stroke Prevention**: Improves cholesterol levels and reduces inflammation.

5. **Fish (Salmon, Cod)**

- **Nutritional Benefits**: Rich in omega-3 fatty acids.
  - **Stroke Prevention**: Lowers blood pressure and triglyceride levels.

6. **Whole Grains (Quinoa, Whole Wheat)**
   - **Nutritional Benefits**: High in fiber, vitamins, and minerals.
   - **Stroke Prevention**: Maintains healthy blood sugar levels and reduces cholesterol.

7. **Legumes (Black Beans, Chickpeas)**

- **Nutritional Benefits**: High in protein, fiber, and essential nutrients.
- **Stroke Prevention**: Helps in managing weight and blood pressure.

8. **Avocado**
   - **Nutritional Benefits**: Rich in healthy fats and potassium.
   - **Stroke Prevention**: Lowers bad cholesterol and maintains healthy blood pressure.

9. **Greek Yogurt**
   - **Nutritional Benefits**: High in protein and probiotics.

- **Stroke Prevention**: Supports gut health and reduces inflammation.

10. **Olive Oil**
   - **Nutritional Benefits**: High in monounsaturated fats and antioxidants.
   - **Stroke Prevention**: Improves heart health and reduces the risk of stroke.

Adhering to this plan provides a balanced intake of nutrients critical for maintaining cardiovascular health and reducing stroke risk. The repetitive nature of the meals ensures ease of preparation while still delivering variety and essential nutrients needed for overall health.

Book Summary

Book Summary: "The Latest Discovery on Stroke Recovery and Prevention Cookbook" by Abraham Hunter

"The Latest Discovery on Stroke Recovery and Prevention Cookbook" by Abraham Hunter is an essential guide that combines scientific research, personal experience, and culinary expertise to address the critical issue of stroke prevention and recovery. This book provides a comprehensive approach to understanding strokes, their causes, and the vital role of nutrition in combating this prevalent health risk.

What is a Stroke?

A stroke is a medical emergency caused by the interruption of blood supply to the brain, leading to potential brain damage. The book delves into the three primary types of strokes:

1. **Ischemic Stroke**: The most common type, resulting from a blocked artery.

2. **Hemorrhagic Stroke**: Caused by a ruptured blood vessel in the brain.

3. **Transient Ischemic Attack (TIA)**: Often referred to as a mini-stroke, it serves as a warning sign for future strokes.

 Historical Context

Hunter traces the history of stroke from its early descriptions by Hippocrates to modern-day medical advancements. This historical perspective highlights the progress made in understanding and treating strokes, providing readers with a context for the current knowledge and strategies outlined in the book.

Personal Insight

Drawing from personal experience of living with a stroke patient, Hunter offers a compassionate and informed perspective on the challenges faced by stroke survivors and their families. This personal touch adds depth and relatability to the book, emphasizing the importance of support and effective care in stroke recovery.

Importance of the Book

With the rising incidence of strokes, this book is timely and crucial. It emphasizes proactive measures to prevent strokes and provides valuable resources for those already affected. Hunter's holistic approach ensures that readers receive well-rounded advice that integrates the latest scientific discoveries with practical solutions.

30-Day Menu Plan

One of the standout features of the book is the 30-day menu plan. This plan is carefully curated to meet the nutritional needs of stroke patients while also being easy to prepare and enjoyable to eat. The recipes focus on ingredients known to support brain health and cardiovascular function, facilitating the recovery process.

Key Learnings

1. **Scientific Insights**: Detailed explanations of stroke mechanisms, risk factors, and the latest prevention strategies.
2. **Nutritional Guidance**: Information on the role of diet in stroke prevention and recovery, highlighting beneficial foods and nutrients.

3. **Lifestyle Advice**: Practical tips for making sustainable lifestyle changes to reduce stroke risk.

4. **Delicious Recipes**: A variety of recipes that are both nutritious and delicious, ensuring stroke patients receive the necessary nutrients without compromising on taste.

5. **30-Day Plan**: A comprehensive guide to meal planning, complete with shopping lists and preparation tips to simplify the process.

Conclusion

"The Latest Discovery on Stroke Recovery and Prevention Cookbook" is more than just a cookbook; it is a vital resource for anyone at risk of stroke, recovering from a stroke, or caring for a stroke patient. It offers a blend of scientific knowledge, personal experience, and practical advice, making it an indispensable tool in the fight against stroke. By following the guidance provided, readers can significantly enhance their quality of life and take meaningful steps towards stroke prevention and recovery.